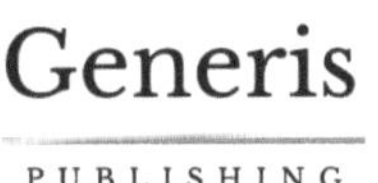

AF448217

Bovine Trypanosomosis in Tsetse Free Adamawa Plateau of Cameroon

Sevidzem Silas Lendzele[1],
Mamoudou Abdoulmoumini[2],
Bouba Mohamadou[2],
Jacques François Mavoungou[3]

Institutions of affiliations:
[1]Ecole Doctorale des Grandes Ecoles de Libreville, Gabon.
[2]Department of Parasitology and Parasitological Desease, School of Veterinary Medicine and Sciences, University of Ngaoundéré, Cameroon.
[3] Institut de recherche en Ecologie Tropicale (IRET-CENAREST), BP : 13354, Libreville, Gabon.

CIP a Camerei Naționale a Cărții

Bovine Trypanosomosis in Tsetse Free Adamawa Plateau of Cameroon / Sevidzem Silas Lendzele, Mamoudou Abdoulmoumini, Bouba Mohamadou, Jacques François Mavoungou. – Chișinău : Generis Publishing, 2020 (Print on demand). – 38 p. : fig., tab.

Referințe bibliogr.: p. 29-34.

ISBN 978-9975-154-39-0.

636.2.093(671.1)

B 74

Cover image: www.pixabay.com

Generis Publishing
Online orders: www.generis-publishing.com
Orders by email: info@generis-publishing.com

TABLE OF CONTENTS

LIST OF FIGURES

LIST OF TABLES

ABSTRACT

African Animal Trypanosomosis (AAT) is an economically important cattle disease in sub-Saharan Africa (SSA) and Cameroon in particular, but no information exists on the role of mechanical vectors in its epizootiology in the tsetse free Adamawa Plateau. A cross sectional survey was conducted for the first time from January to December 2017 at the Ngaoundéré municipal abattoir (receiving cattle from tsetse-infested and tsetse-non infested zones) and Galim rangeland (tsetse free zone) to fill this gap. 739 blood samples from abattoir cattle were collected and examined parasitologically using the Buffy Coat Technique (BCT), whereas fly (n=53) and cattle (n=42) blood samples from Galim were screened for trypanosomes using the nested Polymerase Chain Reaction (nPCR). This study revealed the presence of trypanosomosis in slaughtered cattle with an overall parasitological prevalence of 12.72 % and significantly higher during the rainy season (15.60 %) than in the dry season (10.44 %). *Trypanosoma congolense* (43.62 %) was the predominant trypanosome species infecting the animals and closely followed by *Trypanosoma brucei* (36.17 %), *Trypanosoma vivax* (12.76 %) and mixed infections (7.45 %). A very low parasitaemia (10^2 to 10^3 trypanosomes/ml) was observed in 85% of the infected cattle. The mean packed cell volume (PCV) value of parasitaemic cattle (29.24 %) was lower than that of aparasitaemic cattle (30.05 %). In the 182 cattle with poor Body Condition Score (BCS), 11 % were infected. However, trypanosomosis did not significantly affect PCV and BCS. In Galim, the nPCR showed an overall bovine trypanosomosis of 7%, while 18.9 % of flies tested positive. Also, the nPCR indicated the occurrence of *T. theileri* and *T. vivax* in cattle as well as *T. theileri*, *T. vivax*, and *T. evansi* in tabanids. This study establishes that the presence of trypanosomosis in cattle in Ngaoundéré is possibly spread mechanically by tabanids as well as suggests the possiblility of its introduction in the tsetse free rangeland of Ngaoundere by trade and transhumant cattle.

Keyword: Trypanosomosis, Cattle, Prevalence, Abattoir, Season, Ngaoundéré.

1. INTRODUCTION

Trypanosomosis is a disease caused by a parasite of the genus *Trypanosoma*. African animal trypanosomosis (AAT) is biologically transmitted by tsetse flies of the genus *Glossina* (Sevidzem et al., 2016) and mechanically transmitted by other blood sucking dipterous insect groups (tabanids, stomoxyines, etc.) (Lendzele et al., 2019; Mamoudou et al., 2017). Trypanosoma species such as *T. b. brucei*, *T. vivax*, and *T. congolense* causes AAT in animals while those of the *Trypanosoma brucei* complex such as *T. b. gambiense* and *T. b. rhodesiense* causes Human African Trypanosomosis (HAT) in humans (Simarro et al., 2010). AAT is considered as the main health and production constraint in livestock production in SSA (Swallow, 2000; Shaw et al., 2014). In Cameroon, AAT is ranked among the important cattle diseases that constitute a threat to its livestock industry (Motta et al., 2017). Tsetse fly vectors are present in 8.5 million km^2 in 37 countries, where 46 million cattle are exposed to AAT that directly affect livestock health, agricultural capacity and land use (Alsan, 2015).

The Adamawa region of Cameroon is one of the important cattle rearing regions of the country (MINEPIA, 2013). After the 1994 tsetse erradication campaign, the Adamawa plateau was segmented into three zones consisting of the infested, non-infested and the buffer zones by the Special Mission for Tsetse Eradication (MSEG) to ease control (Mamoudou et al., 2009). Recent reports of AAT in the region shows that the disease still occurs in cattle in the tsetse infested zones with prevalence upto 30 % (Mamoudou et al., 2015a; Mpouam et al., 2011). However, there is no report on the AAT situation in the tsetse free range land of Ngaoundere given that trade cattle from the infested Northern region especially Mayo Rey are brought to cattle markets and abattoirs of such tsetse free areas (**Figure 1**).

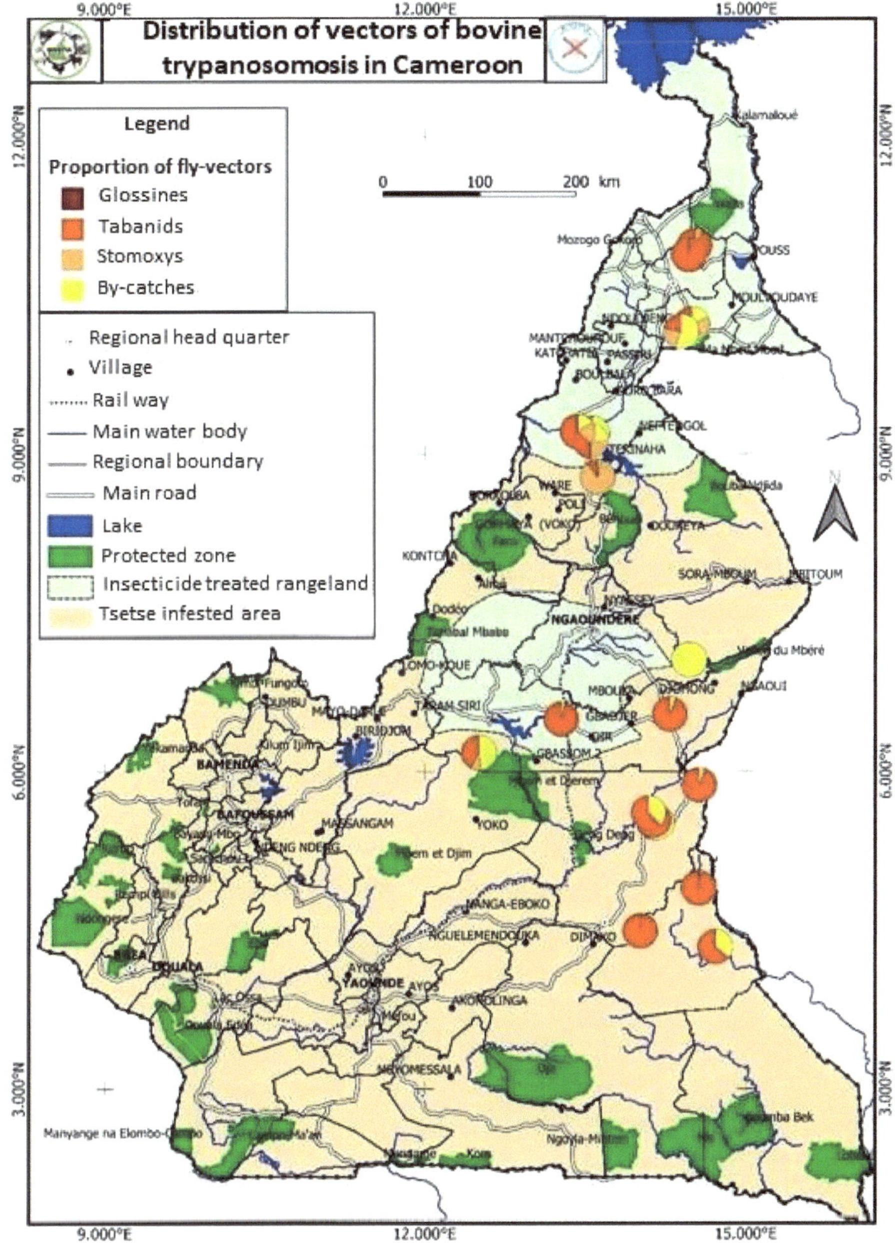

Figure 1 : Map of Cameroon showing bovine trypanosomosis vectors distribution (By MSEG, 2019)

The North region harbours several tsetse pockets with AAT prevalences of 14.3% and 9% reported in the Division of Faro and Mayo-Rey respectively (Achukwi and Musongong, 2009; Mamoudou et al., 2016). Despite enormous resources deployed by the Cameroonian government and breeders to erradicate tsetse and AAT, this parasite remains prevalent in the Adamawa Plateau (Woudamyata, 2014).

The approach used to identify trypanosomes in the Adamawa was by buffy coat technique which is not very sensitive compared to the Polymerase Chain Reaction (PCR), reason why only three species of AAT has been identied in past surveys. However, recent molecular studies by Ngomtcho et al., (2017) and Paguem et al., (2019) to identify *Trypanosoma* species in Adamawa led to the idenfication of *T. grayi* and *T. theileri* in cattle that has not yet been reported in Cameroon.

There is no molecular entomological study that attempts to identify the different *Trypanosom*a species harbored by mechanical vectors such as tabanids and stomoxyines that frequently occur in pasture areas of the Adamawa Plateau (Lendzele et al., 2019). Interestingly, Paguem et al., (2019) reported the widespread of *Trypanosoma* species in Ngaoundere in the absence of tsetse. Additionally, it has been reported that in the absence of tsetse flies, mechanical vectors such as tabanids and stomoxyines can still play a role in trypanosomosis spread (Wells, 1972; Boese et al., 1987; Desquesnes et al., 2003a; Desquesnes et al., 2003b; Taioe et al., 2017).

Although much work has been conducted in several African countries on the prevalence of bovine trypanosomosis at the abattoir level, to the best of our knowledge, no such study has been conducted in Cameroon. Also, no study in the country tried to establish the role of mechanical vectors (tabanids and stomoxyines) in the transmission of trypanosomosis in tsetse free areas. It is in this context that this study was designed with main objective to contribute to a better understanding of the epidemiology of bovine trypanosomosis. Specifically (1) to determine the parasitological and molecular prevalences of trypanosomosis in cattle and mechanical vectors , (2) to show the effect of bovine trypanosomosis on health status of animals, (3) to study the seasonal variation of the infection rate of bovine trypanosomosis, and (4) to trace the origin of the animals that are brought to the Ngaoundere abattoir in order to clearly define the potential source of infection.

2. MATERIALS AND METHODS

2.1. Study area

The study was conducted from January to December 2017 at the Ngaoundere abattoir, located between latitude 7°-8° north and longitude 13°-14° east. Here, approximately 55 cattle are slaughtered daily and most of them originate from Vina division and Mayo Rey division (with past records on mechanical vectors and *Trypanosoma* species occurence) (Mamoudou et al., 2016). The main breeds of cattle encountered in this abattoir include Bokolo, Red Fulani, Gudali x White Fulani, Bokolo x Charolais, and Gudali (Ngu Ngwa et al., 2020). The other sampling site was Galim, a pasture area, located 25 Km from the town of Ngaoundere and found between latitude 07° 11, 887' north and longitude 013° 34, 919' east.

2.2. Study population and sample size determination

The study population consisted of cattle slaughtered at the Ngaoundere Municipal abattoir and sedentary cattle from Galim.

2.3. Sampling criteria

The animals were randomly selected on the basis of their availability and the consent of owners.

The sample size was determined using the following formula:

$$N = \frac{1,96 \times 1,96 \; p(1-p)}{d^2}$$ (Thrusfield, 2007),

N : estimated sample size;

p : known prevalence ;

d : precision of estimation.

An estimated prevalence of 50 % was used with precision level of 5% that resulted in minimum sample size of 384 cattle. We increased the sample size to 739 cattle far above the estimated value to avoid sampling errors.

2.4. Blood collection from cattle

Approximately 3 to 4 ml of blood was collected through the jugular vein into containing Ethylene Diamine Tetra Acetic Acid (EDTA) anticoagulant tubes. The tubes were labelled with the animal number, breed, sex, age, BCS, and origin.

2.5. Determination of breed, age and body condition score of animals

The cattle breed were determined using phenotypic characteristics (Lhoste, 1969). Age was determined by examining the dentition and horn rings. The estimation of age by dentition in cattle was based on the examination of the incisors, according to the criteria described by Dumas and Lhoste (1966) while age determination using the horn rings was conducted following the criteria of Debrot and Constantin (1968). The animals were grouped into 3 age groups such as young (<3 years), adults ([3-8 [) and aged (> 8 years) according Aliyou (2014). The BCS was established on a scale of 0 to 5, after examining the animals by palpation of the lumbar region, as well as by assessing its general appearance following the method proposed by Vall and Bayala (2004). The animals were divided into 3 groups according to their BCS: bad (0 to 2), average (3), and good (4 to 5) according to Aliyou (2014). The origin of animals was the village or division from where they were purchased or raised.

2.6. Parasitological testing of cattle blood for trypanosomes

The collected blood samples were transported to the laboratory in a cooler containing icepacks. Parasitological analyses were conducted within five hours of blood collection using the Murray or Buffy Coat Method (Murray et al. 1977). Briefly, the anticoagulant-containing capillary tubes (EDTA) were filled with 4/5 blood. The tubes were sealed with plasticine at one end and placed in the rotor of the microcentrifuge (Hettich HAEMATOKRIT). The blood was centrifuged at 12,000 revolutions per minute for 5 minutes.

2.7. Determination of the Packed Red Blood Cell Volume (PCV)

The PCV was measured using the hematocrit reader (Hawksley Microhematocrit Reader®). Animals with a PCV less than or equal to 24% were considered anemic, while those with PCV> 24% were declared non-anaemic (Mamoudou et al., 2016).

2.8. Microscopic identification of trypanosomes and determination of parasitaemia

The buffy coat was placed on a slide with coverslip and examined microscopically (Micron optik®) using the x 40 magnification. The preparation was examined for mobile trypanosomes according to the criteria described by

Murray et al. (1977). Trypanosomes are easily recognised by their size and movement where *T. congolense* is small in size, has an affinity for red blood cells and with slow movement. *T. vivax* is larger, rapidly crosses the microscopic field along an almost rectilinear trajectory and stopping occasionally. *T. b. brucei* is similar in size to *T. vivax* and has lively movements but is confined to an area where it often runs in circles. The determination of parasitaemia was made using the score of +1 to +6 (Paris et al., 1982), corresponding to the number of trypanosomes per ml of blood.

2.9.   PCR amplification and sequencing of ITS-1 and Ggapdh

Genomic DNA from the buffy coat was extracted using the Wizard Genomic DNA Purification Kit (Promega, Germany) according to the manufacturer's instructions, and then stored at -20 °C. Generic primers were used in a nested PCR targeting kinetoplastid ITS-1 as described previously (Adams et al., 2006; Ngomtcho et al., 2017; Paguem et al., 2020). Briefly, the first 25 µl volume reaction contained 2 µM of each outer primers (Table 1), 0.2 mM dNTP mix, 0.5 U DreamTaq DNA polymerase (Thermo Scientific, Dreieich, Germany), 1× DreamTaq buffer, and 1 µl of extracted DNA isolates. Water and genomic DNA of *T. brucei*, *T. congolense* or *T. grayi* were added as negative and positive controls, respectively. PCR amplification was carried out as follows: initial denaturation step at 95°C for 60 s, followed by 30 amplification cycles with 94°C for 60 s, 52°C for 60 s, 72°C for 30 s, and final extension 72°C for 5 min. After that, the second PCR reaction was carried out with 1 µl of first 1:80 diluted PCR template under the same cycling conditions as described above, except an annealing temperature of 54°C, and using the inner primer pairs (Table 1). 20 µl of the resulting PCR product was loaded onto a 2% TBE/agarose gel stained with 0.5 µg/ml of SERVA DNA Stain G (SERVA, Heidelberg, Germany) and results for *Trypanosoma* species detection read following table 2. Positive PCR amplicons of variable fragment sizes representing different trypanosome species were randomly selected for Sanger sequencing. For those samples, the second reaction was carried out with the total volume of 50 µl and 2 µl of 80-fold diluted first PCR product was used.

An approximately 900 bp region of the glycosomal glyceraldehyde phosphate dehydrogenase (gGAPDH) gene was amplified by nested PCR and sequenced using the primers described in table 1. Nested PCR was carried out using 2xRed Mastermix (Genaxxon Bioscience, Ulm, Germany) to generate PCR products for direct sequencing. In short, first PCR reactions with a final volume of 25 µl contained 1xMastermix, 0.5 µM of outer primers, and 2 µl of genomic DNA template under the following conditions: initial denaturation at 95°C for 3 min, 30 cycles of 95°C for 1 min, annealing at 55°C for 30 s, elongation at 72°C for 1 min, followed by a final elongation step at 72°C for 10 min. The first PCR products were diluted 80-fold and 2 µl was transferred to the second PCR reaction with the inner primers (Table 1) under the same conditions as the first reaction. Amplified products were subjected to electrophoresis on 2 % agarose gels. From the positive PCR products, DNA concentrations were determined on a Nanodrop 1000 (Thermo Scientific, Dreiech, Germany) and sent for sequencing (Macrogen, Netherlands).

Next, positive amplicons were excised from the gel and purified using GeneJet Gel Extraction Kit (Thermo Scientific, Dreiech, Germany) according to the manufacturer's recommendation. DNA concentrations were measured before submitting them to a commercial sequencing provider (Macrogen).

Table 1: Generic Primers used for PCR amplification

Primers	5'- 3' sequence	sequence length	Reference
ITS1-OutF	CTT TGC TGC GTT CTT		
ITS1-OutR	TGC AAT TAT TGG TCG CGC		Adams *et al.*, 2006
ITS1-InF	TAG AGG AAG CAA AAG	(640-180) bp	
ITS1-InR	AAG CCA AGT CAT CCA TCG		
gGAPDH-OutF	TTY GCC GYA TYG GYC GCA TGG		Hamilton *et al.*, 2004
gGAPDH-OutR	ACM AGR TCC ACC ACR CGG TG	900bp	
gGAPDH-InF	CGC GGA TCC ASG GYC TYM TCG GBA MKG AGA T		
gGAPDH-InR	GTT YTG CAG SGT CGC CTT GG		

Primer. In: Inner primer. F: forward. R: reverse.

Table 2: Trypanosome ITS-1 amplicon sizes

Trypanosomes species	Amplicon size (bp)
T. congolense savannah	640
T. congolense riverine/forest	662
T. congolense kilifi	562
T. brucei brucei	426
T. brucei rhodesiense	426
T. brucei gambiense	426
T. avensi	400
T. godfreyi	300
T. vivax	180 and 250
T. theileri	320-
T. grayi	318

Source : Ngomtcho et al., (2017) and Paguem et al., (2019)

2.10. Fly collection

Fly trapping at Galim in Ngaoundere was conducted at the end of the rainy season (October to December) using a Vavoua trap (constructed by Laveissière et Grebaut, 1990) (**Figure 2**). Among the tsetse traps, Vavoua is the cheapest and efficient for the capture of Muscidae especially Stomoxys (Sevidzem and Mavoungou, 2019).

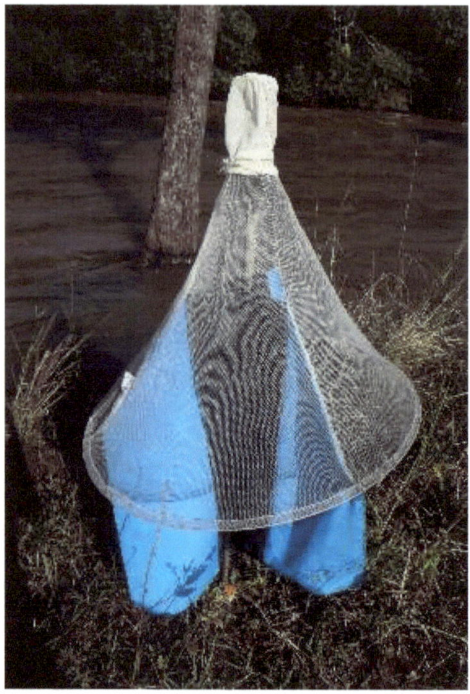

Figure 2 : Vavoua trap (Photo by Sevidzem)

2.11. Fly identification

The identification of tabanids was conducted using the key specimens from West Africa by Desquesnes et al., (2005). The identification of Stomoxys was conducted using the abdominal landmarks prepared by Zumpt (1973) as well as the Central African key for some species by Sevidzem in 2015 (unpublished).

2.12. Data analysis

The prevalence was obtained by using the following formula :

$$\text{Prevalence} = \frac{\text{Number of positive animals sampled}}{\text{Number of animals sampled}} \times 100 \text{ (Thrusfield, 2007)}$$

Statistical analysis was conducted using the XLSTAT version 19.4 statistical software. The Chi-square test of independence and the kruskal-Wallis test were used to compare prevalence rates with associated risk factors. The degrees of significance of all satistical tests were kept at p < 0.05.

3. RESULTS

3.1. Prevalence with origin of slaughtered cattle

Seven hundred and thirty nine (739) cattle were sampled, including 412 in the dry season (January to March) and 327 in the rainy season (May-June). These animals came from 14 cattle markets notably Dang, Dibi, Djalingo, Galdi, Likok, Mbe, Ngaoundere, Tchabal, Tello located in the Vina division and others from Goprey, Mbaka, Touboro, Vogzom, and Yoko, found in the Mayo Rey division. About 55 % of these animals originated from the Mayo Rey division (n=406) and 45 % from the Vina division (n=333). The prevalence with respect to the divisions of origin indicates that higher cases were encountered in animals from Mayo Rey than those from Vina division (**Figure 3**).

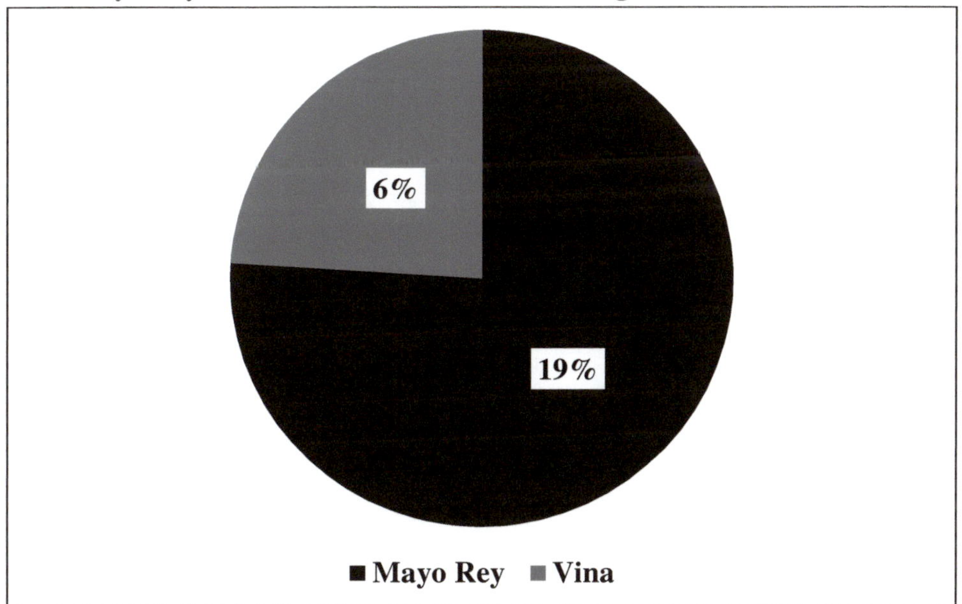

Figure 3: Parasitological prevalence with respect to division of origin

3.2. Prevalence of bovine trypanosomosis at the Ngaoundere Abattoir

Of the 739 cattle sampled, parasitological examination revealed 94 positive samples with parasitological prevalence rate of 12.72% (95% CI: [10.32% - 15.12%]).

3.3. *Trypanosoma* species identified via BCT

The trypanosome species encountered included *T. congolense, T. brucei, T. vivax,* and their mixed infections. The predominance of *T. congolense* (43.62%: 41/94) was observed, followed by *T. brucei* (36.17%: 34/94) and finally *T. vivax* (12.76%: 12/94). In addition to these monospecific infections, mixed infections were recorded, including *T. congolense + T. brucei* (5.32%: 5/94), *T. congolense + T. vivax* (1.06%: 1/94), and *T. congolense + T. brucei + T. vivax* (1.06%: 1/94). The difference between trypanosome species infection rates was significant (p <0.05).

3.4. Association of *Trypanosoma* species and parasitaemia on number of cases

The number of infected animals depended on the *Trypanosoma* infection states (monospecies and polyspecies) (Table 3). Highest number of cases were recorded in animals with the lowest parasitaemia (Table 3).

Table 3: The association of *Trypanosoma* species and parasitaemia on number of cases

Factor		Number	P-value
***Trypanosoma* spp.**	Tb	34	
	Tc	41	
	Tv	12	
	Tb+Tc	5	
	Tc+Tv	1	
	Tb+Tc+Tv	1	0.458
Parasitaemia	10^2 to 10^4	80	
	10^3 to 10^4	12	
	5×10^3 to 5×10^4	2	0.245

Tc=*Trypanosoma congolense*, Tv=*Trypanosoma vivax*, Tb=*Trypanosoma brucei*.

3.5. Prevalence with respect to season

The parasitological prevalence of bovine trypanosomosis with season showed that higher cases were diagnosed in the rainy season than in the dry with a statistically significant difference (p <0.05) (Table 4).

Table 4: Prevalence of trypanosomes with respect to season

Season	Number	Positive	Prevalence (%)	CI (%)
Dry (Jauary to March)	412	43	10.44[a]	[7.49 – 13.39]
Rainy (May to June)	327	51	15.60[b]	[11.18 – 18.94]

Different letters of the alphabet indicate a statistically significatn difference (p < 0,05) at the 95 % confidence interval.

3.6. Prevalence with breed, sex, age and season

In the dry season it was noticed that the Bokolo cattle breed recorded the highest prevalence rate. In this same period, malc cattle recorded the highest prevalence rate. The age cohort with the highest prevalence rate was 3 to 8 years. For the rainy season, the Gudali cattle breed recorded the highest prevalence rate. In the rainy season, Males had a higher infection rate than their female counterparts and the age cohort with the highest prevalence rate consisted of those < 3 years old (Table 5).

Table 5: Prevalence with breed, sex, age and season

Season	Risk factors		Number	Positive	Prevalence (%)	P-value
dry	breed	Akou	150	13	8.67	
(January to March)		Bokolo	3	1	33.33	
		Djafoun	118	14	11.86	
		Goudali	131	14	10.69	
		Metis	10	1	10	0.487
	Sex	Female	368	37	10.05	
		Male	44	6	13.64	0.463
	Age	< 3	14	1	7.14	
		[3-8[	351	39	11.11	
		≥ 8	47	3	6.38	0.701
rainy (May to June)	breed	Akou	81	11	13.58	
		Bokolo	18	2	11.11	
		Djafoun	45	5	11.11	
		Goudali	166	32	19.28	
		Métis	17	1	5.88	0.496
	Sex	Female	299	45	15.05	
		Male	28	6	21.43	0.374
	Age	< 3	21	4	19.05	
		[3-8[	212	32	15.09	
		≥ 8	94	15	15.96	0.821

3.7. Influence of bovine trypanosomosis on hematocrit

Of the 96 animals with hematocrit less than or equal to 24, only 11 (11.46%) had bovine trypanosomosis. In the dry season, 20.93% (9/43) of trypanosomosis-positive animals had haematocrit lower or equal to 24, while in the rainy season only 3.92% (2/51) positive animals had haematocrits less than or equal to 24 (Table 6).

Table 6: Bovine trypanosomosis with haematocrit and sampling seasons

Season	PCV	Number	Positive	Negative	P-value
Dry (January to March)	PCV ≤ 24	77	9	68	
	PCV > 24	335	34	301	0.690
rainy (May to June)	PCV ≤ 24	19	2	17	
	PCV > 24	308	49	259	0.530

3.8.   The influence of bovine trypanosomosis on BCS

Based on the Body Condition Score (BCS) of the animals, only 21.28% (20/94) of trypanosomosis-positive cases were identified to exhibit a poor body condition. These 20 (10.99%) trypanosomosis-positive poor condition animals were inferior to animals with medium and good body conditions and infected with trypanosomes (74: 13.28%). This difference was not statistically significant (p = 0.420). In the dry season (Table 7) the medium BCS animals were the most infected (12.5%) compared to poor BCS animals (2.5) and this difference was statistically significant (p <0.05). In the rainy season, the most infected animals (17.65%) were those with a poor BCS while those with medium BCS were least infected.

Table 7: Influence of BCS on prevalence in the sampling seasons

Season	BCS	Number	Positive	Negative	Prevalencce (%)	P-value
dry (January to March)	Poor (0 to 2)	80	2	78	2.5	
	Medium (3)	329	41	288	12.46	
	Good (4 to 5)	3	0	3	0	0.028
rainy (May to June)	Poor (0 to 2)	102	18	84	17.65	
	Medium (3)	219	32	187	14.61	
	Good (4 to 5)	6	1	5	16.67	0.782

3.9. The apparent density of flies in Galim

The entomological prospection resulted in 127 flies grouped under two families notably Tabanidae and Stomoxyidae. For Tabanidae, two genera were identified- *Chrysops* (deer flies), *Tabanus* (horse flies) and *Haematopota* (clegs) with *Chrysops* highly represented. For the stomoxyines, only one genus was identified and was *Stomoxys*. The apparent density (ADT) of the different fly species was recorded, *C. longicornis* (1.2 flies/trap and day), *H. decora* (0.6 flies/trap and day), *T. taeniola* (0.5 flies /trap and day), *T. gratus* (0.3 flies/trap and day), *S. niger niger* (3.0 flies/trap and day), *S. omega* (0.8 flies/trap and days), *S. niger bilineatus* (0.4 flies per trap and day) and *S. inornatus* (0.2 flies per trap and day) (**Figure 4**).

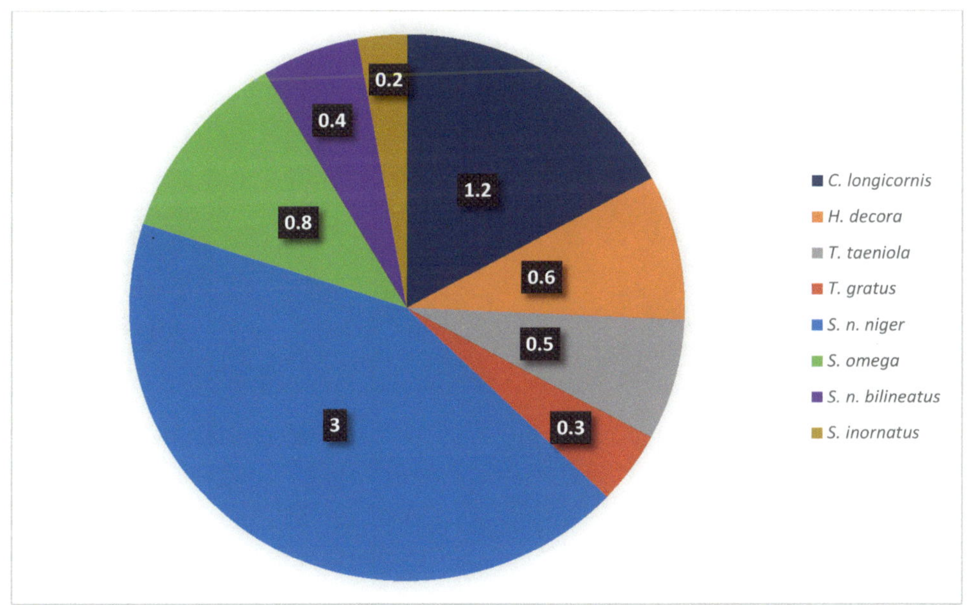

Figure 4: Trap apparent densities of flies caught

3.10. Molecular detection of trypanosomes in cattle

Trypanosoma theileri (3.8%) and *T. vivax* (2.4%) were molecularly detected with an overall molecular prevalence of 7% (**Figure 5 and 6**).

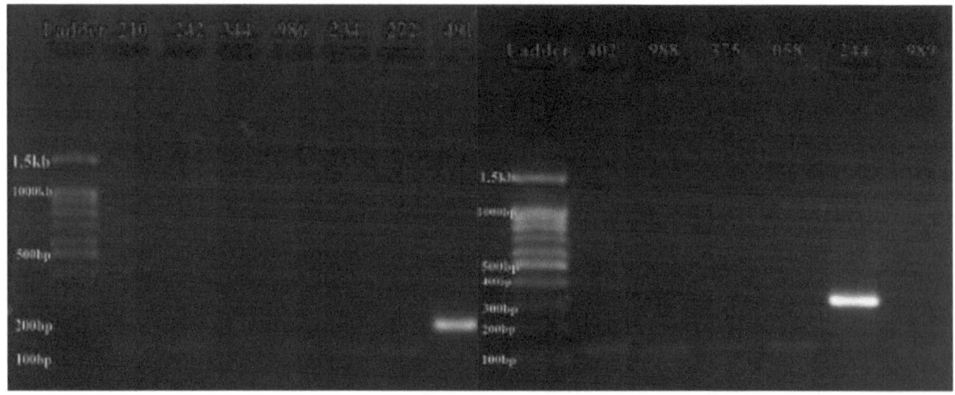

Figure 5: Gel electrophoresis showing signals of *T. theileri* (animal 491) and *T. vivax* (animal 244). Numbers on each sample lane are codes of the sampled cattle.

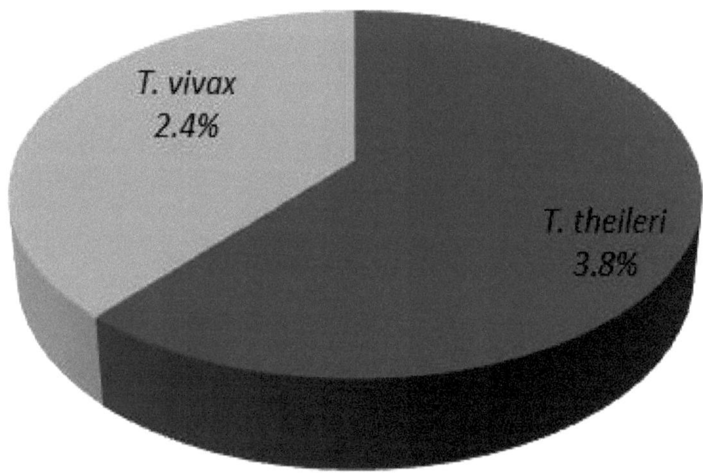

Figure 6: *Trypanosoma* species from screened cattle.

Of the 127 flies caught, 53 of them were screened and 10 positive cases recorded, resulting in an overall fly infection rate of 18.9%. One mix infection of *T. evansi* and *T. theileri*, occurred in *C. longicornis* (**Figure 7**).

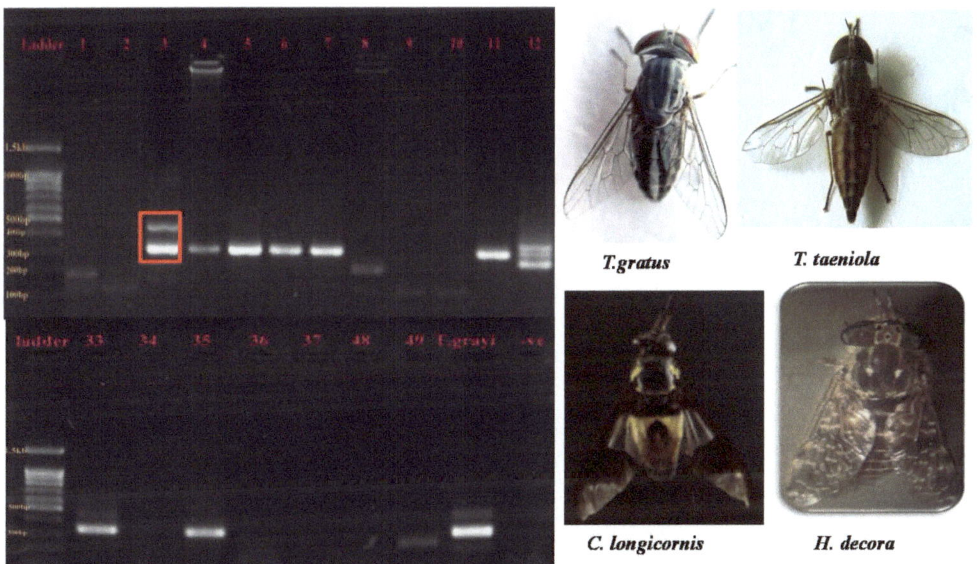

Figure 7: Gel electrophoresis showing signals of Trypanosoma species. The numbers on each sample lane are codes of the screened flies. Lane 3 is *C. longicornis* with mix infection (*T. theileri + T. evansi*) indicated with red rectangle; lane 8 and 11 shows *H. decora* with single infection (*T. theileri*); lanes 5, 6, 7, 33, 35 indicates *C. longicornis* single infection (*T. theileri*) and lane 12 shows *T. gratus* single infection (*T. theileri*).

It was noticed that *C. longicornis* harbored all the *Trypanosoma* species identified in the present study. *H. decora*, *T. taeniola* and *T. gratus* harbored only *T. theileri* (**Table 8**). All the *Stomoxys* species screened were negative for trypanosomes.

Table 8: Flies caught/screened and the Trypanosoma species identified in flies

Species	Number	screened	nPCR	nPCR (%)	*Trypanosoma* species identified		
					T. theileri	*T. vivax*	*T. evansi*
C. longicornis	21	21	3	14.3	++	+	+
H. decora	10	9	5	55.6	+++++	-	-
T. taeniola	9	7	1	14.3	+	-	-
T. gratus	6	4	1	25	+	-	-
S. n. niger	52	8	0	0	-	-	-
S. omega	14	2	0	0	-	-	-
S. n. bilineatus	8	1	0	0	-	-	-
S. inornatus	7	1	0	0	-	-	-
Total	127	53	10		9	1	1

+ indicates a case, - indicates negative, nPCR: nested polymerase chain reaction.

DISCUSSION

3.12. Prevalence of *Trypanosoma* species and host related factors in Ngaoundere Abattoir

The abattoir survey in Ngaoundere indicated the presence of trypanosomosis in cattle with parasitological prevalence of 12.72%. This result is superior to that reported by Mpouam et al. (2011) in the Vina and by Mamoudou et al., (2016) in Mayo-Rey with prevalence rates of 11.5% and 9% respectively. This difference may be due to the fact that the animals slaughtered at the Ngaoundéré municipal abattoir originated from bovine trypanosomosis endemic areas such as Mayo-Rey with highest number of cattle recorded in the Ngaoundere abattoir. Conversely, this result is less than 29.4%, obtained in Almé in the Faro and Déo division (Mamoudou et al., 2015a). This difference may be due to the nature of study areas in terms of tsetse fly infestation, where Almé is a tsetse infested area and no vector control has never been conducted as compared to Vina with continuous and intensive ongoing vector control. It was interesting to know that those animals coming from the Mayo Rey division were highly infected with trypanosomosis than those from the Vina Division. This finding was not suprising because Mayo Rey harbors dense tsetse and tabanids pockets as already reported (Sevidzem et al., 2016 ; Mamoudou et al., 2016 ; Lendzele et al., 2017) that could be implicated in transmission as compared to Vina division with no reports on tsetse infestation (Lendzele et al., 2019). Regarding season, the prevalence is significantly higher in the rainy season (15.60%) compared to the dry season (10.44%), probably due to highest tsetse and other fly vectors densities occuring during this season in the Plateau of Adamawa (Sevidzem et al., 2015). This increase in prevalence during the rainy season corroborates the results obtained in Mayo-Rey by Mamoudou et al. (2015b). In the present study, *T. congolense* was the predominant species. The predominance of this species has already been reported by Tanenbe et al. (2010) in the Faro and Deo and vina (Adamawa Region) divisions by Achukwi and Musongong (2009). This indicates that there is contact between the animals and tsetse flies and other biting dipterous insects that could lead to high transmission in those areas (Hoaré, 1977). The very low parasitaemias observed in this present study is similar to that reported by Mpouam et al. (2011). This result reflects the regular use of trypanocides by farmers in breeding areas (OIE, 2013). The highest parasitaemia levels (5×10^3 to 5×10^4) were observed in infections caused by *T. congolense*. This observation is consistent with that of Mpouam et al. (2011) and could be explained by the fact that *T. congolense* is the most pathogenic species for cattle (OIE, 2005).

The average hematocrit of the animals was 30.09 and did not differ from the 30.2% obtained in Vina (Mpouam et al., 2011). The proportion of individuals with hematocrit less than 24 was higher in the dry season (18.69%) than in the rainy season (5.81%). This increase in mean hematocrit in the rainy season was also recorded by Ogunsanmi et al. (2010) and Mamoudou et al. (2016). This may be as a result of increased pasture availability associated with increased nutrient values during the rainy season (Ogunsanmi et al., 2010, Deffo et al., 2011). No endogenous factor (sex, age and breed) considered had a significant influence on the prevalence of bovine trypanosomosis at the Ngaoundere municipal abattoir and this observation was similar to that made by other authors (Achukwi and Musongong, 2009, Eyasu and Ahmed, 2013 and Mamoudou et al. 2015a).

The mean hematocrit of positive animals for trypanosomosis was lower than that of negative animals. This decrease in mean hematocrit in positive animals was significant during the dry season. Several authors have reported a decrease in mean hematocrit in animals infected with trypanosomiasis (Mamoudou et al.,

2016, Mamoudou et al., 2015b). This result can be explained by the fact that bovine trypanosomiasis causes a sharp decrease in the number of red blood cells, resulting in a drop in the hematocrit. The scarcity of pasture and stress related to the search of food during the dry season, might have contributed to the poor body condition of the animals during this period. The influence of trypanosome species and degree of parasitaemia were not significant in trypanosomosis-positive animals. However, mean hematocrit was lower in cattle infected with *T. congolense* and especially in cattle with mixed infections caused by *T. congolense* + *T. vivax*, and *T. congolense* + *T. brucei*. These results are similar to those obtained by Mamoudou et al. (2015c) and could be explained by the fact that *T. congolense* is the most pathogenic species of cattle (OIE, 2005) and its presence in the host system greatly reduces its red blood cell count. Only 11.46% of animals with a hematocrit less than or equal to 24 had trypanosomosis, hence the existence of other factors or anaemia-causing diseases such as gastrointestinal helminthosis (Moti et al., 2013), haemoparasites, ectoparasites (ticks) (Abah et al., 2019) and nutritional deficiencies (Mamoudou et al., 2016) cannot be rolled-out. Several studies have shown that animals parasitized by both trypanosomes and helminths recorded lower hematocrit compared to animals with a single infection (Mamoudou et al., 2015d, Moti et al., 2013).

Of a total of 182 poor BCS animals, only 20 of them were trypanosomosis positive. These 20 trypanosomosis-positive poor BCS animals were inferior to animals (n=74) with medium and good BCS infected with trypanosomosis. This result is different from that obtained by Samdi et al. (2011) in a study conducted at the Kaduna abattoir in Nigeria. The decrease in the BCS could be partially linked to *Trypanosoma* species infection as well as other factors including gastrointestinal helminthosis, ectoparasitosis, haemoparasitosis transmitted by ticks, stress and nutritional deficiencies during the dry season (Mamoudou et al., 2016).

3.13. Molecular prevalence of *Trypanosoma* species in cattle and mechanical vectors in Ngaoundere

The occurrence of tabanids and stomoxyines, mechanical vectors of bovine trypanosomosis in the pasture area of Ngaoundere is an indication of the risk of transmission of the disease in the absence of glossines. In the Far north region of Cameroon, there are no tsetse flies but the area is heavily infested by tabanids and stomoxyines. In the Far north region of Cameroon, Suh et al., (2017) reported the occurrence of *T. vivax* indicating the important role of mechanical vectors in transmission. The present study identified one species of the genus *Chrysops* (*Chrysops longicornis*), one species of the genus *Haematopota* (*Haematopota decora*), two species of *Tabanus* (*Tabanus taeniola* and *Tabanus gratus*) and four species of *Stomoxys* (*S. n. niger*, *S. omega*, *S. n. bilineatus* and *S. inornatus*). *C. longicornis* was infected with all the screened *Trypanosoma* species (*T. theileri*, *T. vivax* and *T. evansi*), but the positive cases of *H. decora*, *T. taeniola* and *T. gratus* were only from *T. theileri*. Additionally, *H. decora* was frequently contaminated with *T. theileri* as compared to any other infected fly. These findings were not surprising as Taioe et al., (2017) already reported that some members of the genera-*Tabanus*, *Haematopota*, *Philoliche*, *Atylotus* and *Ancala* were positive for trypanosomes. Similarly, Boese et al., (1987) reported the cyclical transmission of *T. theileri* by *Haematopota* species. The overall molecular prevalence of trypanosomes in cattle was 7% and was caused by *T. theileri* and *T. vivax*. These trypanosomes have been reported to be transmitted cyclically and acyclically (Boese et al., 1987; Desquesnes et al., 2003a). There was no *T. evansi* detected in cattle samples of the sampled animals. This could be explained by the fact that wild animals such as monkeys present in the area as well as cattle from neighbouring Dawa Ranch and Centre Zootechnique could be reservoir host fo *T. evansi*. Futhermore, the presence of Camels in Ngaoundere might be a source of contamination of local cattle breeds with *T. evansi* since camels are natural reservoir host of this species (Lun and Brun, 1992). The absence of positive cases of trypanosomes in *Stomoxys* could be explained by the low number of samples screened in the present study and not their incapability to harbour trypanosomes. *Stomoxys* species have been shown to be implicated in the mechanical transmission of *T. evansi* and *T. congolense* (Sumba et al., 1997).

4. CONCLUSION

From the abattoir survey, the parasitological prevalence was 12.72%. This prevalence was significantly higher in the rainy season than in the dry season and *Trypanosoma congolense* was the most frequent species. Infected cattle had lower hematocrit values than uninfected cattle. Poor body condition animals were highly infected with this parasite. This study confirms the presence of trypanosomosis in cattle slaughtered in Ngaoundere and indicates that high risk could be from cattle coming from the tsetse infested Mayo Rey division in the North region. The nested PCR showed the presence of *T. theileri* and *T. vivax* in cattle as well as *T. theileri*, *T. vivax* and *T. evansi* in tabanids in the tsetse free belt and trypanosomosis hypo-endemic rangeland of Galim. Therefore the role of Tabanidae in the epizootiology of bovine trypanosomosis in tsetse free areas of Cameroon should not be neglected.

5. REFERENCES

Achukwi MD, Musongong GA. 2009. Trypanosomosis in the Doayo/Namchi (*Bos taurus*) and zebu White Fulani (*Bos indicus*) cattle in Faro Division, North Cameroon. Journal of Applied Biosciences, 15, 80 - 814.

Abah S, Abel W, Njan Nlôga AM, Lendzele SS, Mamoudou A, Dickmu S, Poueme NRS, Aboubakar Y, Zoli A, Christian N, Souley A. 2019. Tick infestation and haematocrit alteration of cattle in Boklé-Garoua (Northern Cameroon). International Journal of Current Research in Bioscience and Plant Biology, 6(11), 29-34.

Aliyou H. 2014. Etude épidémiologique de la trypanosomose bovine dans le Mayo-rey région du nord Cameroun. In Mémoire présenté en vue de l'obtention du diplôme de docteur en médecine vétérinaire. Ecole des sciences et de médecine vétérinaire, Université de Ngaoundéré, Cameroun, 104 pages.

Alsan M. 2015. The effect of the TseTse Fly on African Development. American Economic review, 105, 382-410.

Boese R, Friedhoff KT, Olbrich S, Büscher G, Domeyer I. 1987. Transmission of Trypanosoma theileri to cattle by Tabanidae. Parasitology Research, 73, 421–424.

Dayo G.-K. 2004. Contribution à l'identification de marqueurs génétiques de tolérance/sensibilité des bovins aux trypanosomoses. In Memoire de DEA de Biologie Animale, Université Cheick Anta Diop de Dakar, Sénégal. 68 pages.

De La Rocque S, Cuisance D. 2005. La Tsé-tsé, une mouche singulière et dangereuse. Insectes, 136 (1). 27-31.

De La Rocque, S. & Dia, M.L. 2001. Les moyens de lutte contre la trypanosomose animale. In Utilisation des trypanocides en Afrique Sub-saharienne. Actes du séminaire sous régional tenu du 06 au 09 février 2001. Ecole Inter - Etats des Sciences et Médecine Vétérinaires. Université Cheikh Anta Diop de Dakar, Sénégal. 170 pages.

De La Rocque, S. 2003. Epidémiologie des trypanosomoses africaines, analyse et prévision du risque dans des paysages en transformation. Courrier de l'environnement de l'INRA. 49, 80-86.

Deffo V, Tendonkeng-Pamo E, Tchotsoua M, Lieugomg M, Arene C, Nwagbo EC. 2011. Determination of the best forage production period for cattle farming in the Adamawa Region of Cameroon. International Journal of Biological and Chemical Sciences, 4(1), 130-44.

Desquesnes M, Dia ML. 2003a. Mechanical transmission of *Trypanosoma congolense* in cattle by the African tabanid *Atylotus agrestis*. Experimental parasitology, 105, 226-231.

Desquesnes M, Dia ML. 2003b. *Trypanosoma vivax*: mechanical transmission in cattle by one of the most common African tabanids, *Atylotus agrestis*. Experimental Parasitology, 103 (1-2), 35–43.

Desquesnes M, Dia M L, Acapovi G, Yoni W. 2005. Les vecteurs mécaniques des trypanosomoses animales.-CIRDES.-Bobo-Dioulasso, Burkina Faso.

Eyasu A, Ahmed Y. 2013. Prevalence of bovine trypanosomiasis in Wolaita zone kindokoish District of Ethiopia. African Journal of Agricultural Research, 8(49), 6383-6387.

Hoare CA. 1972. The trypanosomes of Mammals. A Zoological Monograph. Blackwell, Oxford, 102-134.

Hoste CH, Chalon E, d'Ieteren G, Trail JCM. 1988. Le bétail trypanotolérant en Afrique Occidentale et Centrale, vol. 3: Bilan d'une décennie, Etude FAO: Production et Sante Animales. 20/3. 217 pages.

Lendzele SS, Mamoudou A, Yao-Acapovi GL. Spatial repartition of tabanids in different zones of north Cameroon. Biodiversity International Journal, 1(2), 00010. DOI:10.15406/bij.2017.01.00010.

Lendzele SL, Eisenbarth A, Zinga-Koumba RC, Mavoungou JF, Renz A. 2019. Aspects of the bionomics of hematophagous symbovine dipterans in a hyperinfested rangeland of Ngaoundere (Adamawa-Cameroon). Journal of Asia-Pacific Entomology, 22, 1019–1030.

Lhoste P. 1969. Les races bovines de l'Adamaoua (Cameroun). Institut d'élevage et de Médecine vétérinaire des pays tropicaux, Edition ORSTOM. 19 pages.

Lun ZR, Brun R GW.1992. Kinetoplast DNA and molecular karyotypes of Trypanosoma evansi and Trypanosoma equiperdum from China. Molecular Biochemistry and Parasitology, 50(2), 189-196. PMID: 1311051.

Mamoudou A, Zoli A, Van den Bossche P, Delespaux V, D. Cuisance, Geerts S. 2009. Half a Century of Tsetse and Animal Trypanosomosis Control on the Adamawa Plateau in Cameroon. Revue d'Élevage et de Médecine vétérinaire des Pays Tropicaux, 62 (1) : 33-38.

Mamoudou A, Sevidzem SL, Feussom JM, Mfewou A. 2017. Evaluation of efficacy of Deltamethrin 10%-impregnated screens in a tsetse endemic area in the Sudano-Sahelian region of Cameroon.

Mamoudou A, Ebene NJ, Fongho SP, Mfopit MY. 2015b. Prevalence and impact of bovine trypanosomiasis in Mayo Rey division, a Soudano-Sahelian zone of Cameroon. Journal of Parasitology and Vector Biology, 7(5), 80-88.

Mamoudou A, Fongho SP, Ebene NJ. 2015d. Trypanosomes and helminths infections in Mayo Rey Division of Cameroon and impact of concurrent infections on cattle. Journal of Veterinary Medicine and Animal Health, 7(6), 215-220.

Mamoudou A, Njanloga A, Aliyou H, Fongho SP, Achukwi MD. 2016. Animal trypanosomosis in clinically healthy cattle of north Cameroon: epidemiological implications. Parasites & Vectors, 9, 206, 8 pages.

Mamoudou A, Payne VK, Sevidzem SL. 2015a. Current prevalence of cattle trypanosomiasis and of its vector in Alme, the infested zone of Adamawa plateau Cameroon, two decades after the tsetse eradication campaign. International Journal of Biological and Chemical Sciences. 9(3), 1588-1598.

Mamoudou A, Payne VK, Sevidzem SL. 2015c. Hematocrit alterations and its effects in naturally infected indigenous cattle breeds due to

Trypanosoma spp. on the Adamawa Plateau – Cameroon. Veterinary World, 8(22), 813-818.

MINEPIA, 'Ministère de l'Elevage, des Pêches et des Industries Animales', MINEPIA Policy Document. 2013, 29.

Mpouam SE, Achukwi MD, Feussom KJM, Bengaly Z, Ouedraogo GA. 2011. Serological and parasitological prevalence of bovine trypanosomosis in small holder farms of the Vina division, Adamawa region of Cameroon. Journal of Parasitology and Vector Biology, 3 (4), 44-51.

Ngomtcho SCH, Weber J, Ngo Bum E, Terlumu GT, Kelm S, Achukwi MD. 2017. Molecular screening of tsetse flies and cattle reveal different *Trypanosoma* species including *T. grayi* and *T. theileri* in northern Cameroon. Parasite & Vectors, 10, 631.

Ngu-Ngwa V, Bessong TNA, Ndukum JA. 2020. Seroprevalence and Risk Factors of Leptospirosis among slaughtered Cattle and Abattoir Workers in Ngaoundéré, Cameroon. Asian Journal of Research in Animal and Veterinary Sciences, 5(1), 8-19.

Ogunsanmi AO, Ikede BO, Akpavies O. 2000. Effects of management, season, vegetation zone and breed on the prevalence of bovine trypanosomiasis in southwestern Nigeria. Israel Journal of Veterinary Medicine, 55 (2), 69-73.

OIE 2005. Manuel terrestre de l'OIE. In: Manuel terrestre de l'OIE, 644-652.

OIE 2013. Diagnostic techniques. In Terrestrial manual, Chapter 2.4.17. Trypanosomosis (tsetse-transmitted), 11 pages.

Paguem A, Babette A, Dieudonné N, Judith SW, Ngomtcho SCH, Kingsley TM, Mamoudou A, Eisenbarth A, Renz A, Sørge K, Mbunkah DA. 2019. Widespread co-endemicity of *Trypanosoma* species infecting cattle in the Sudano-sahelian and Guinea Savannah zones of Cameroon. BMC Veterinary Research, 15:344.

Paris J, Murray M, Mcodimba F. 1982. A comparative evaluation of the parasitological techniques currently available for the diagnosis of African trypanosomiasis in cattle. Acta Tropica, 39, 307-316.

Samdi SM, Fajinmi AO, Kalejaye JO, Wayo B, Haruna MK, Yarnap JE.2011. Prevalence of Trypanosomosis in Cattle at Slaughter in Kaduna Central Abattoir. Asian Journal of Animal Sciences, 5 (2), 162-165.

Sevidzem SL, Mavoungou JF. 2019. Relative Efficacy of Tsetse Traps and Live Cattle in Estimating the Real Abundance of Blood-Sucking Insects. Journal of Applied Sciences, 19, 690-700.

Sevidzem SL, Mamoudou A, Acapovi-Yao GL, Achiri M, Tchuinkam T, Zinga-Koumba CR, Mavoungou JF. 2016. First Inventory of Non-biting and Bitting Muscids of North Cameroon. International Research Journal of Biological Science, 5(10), 12-20.

Sevidzem SL, Raymond T, Zinga-Koumba R, Mamoudou A, Ndjonka D, Mavoungou JF. 2019. Insecticide coated screen models reduce insect-vector population in a pasture area in Ngaoundere, Cameroon. Trends in Applied Science Research, 14, 80-89.

Sevidzem SL, Mamoudou A, Woudamyata AF, Zoli PA. 2015. Contribution to the knowledge of Eco-diversity and density of tsetse (Glossinidae) and other biting flies (Tabanidae and Stomoxyinae) in the fly controlled-infested livestock/wild life interface of the Adamawa plateau-Cameroon. Journal of Entomology and Zoology Studies, 3(5), 329-333.

Shaw AP, Cecchi G, Wint GR, Mattioli RC, Robinson TP. 2014. Mapping the economic benefits to livestock keepers from intervening against bovine trypanosomosis in Eastern Africa. Preventive Veterinary Medicine, 113, 197-210.

Simarro PP, Cecchi G, Paone M, Franco JR, Diarra A. 2010. The Atlas of human African trypanosomiasis: a contribution to global mapping of neglected tropical diseases. International Journal of Health, 9, 57.

Suh PF, Njiokou F, Mamoudou A, Ahmadou TM, Mouhaman A, Garabed R. 2017. Bovine trypanosomiasis in tsetse-free pastoral zone of the Far-North region, CameroonJ Vector Borne Disease, 54, 263-269.

Sumba AL 1997. Mechanical transmission of *T. evansi* and *T. congolense* by African *Stomoxys* spp. A thesis submitted in partial fulfillment for the degree of Master of Science (Medical and Veterinary Parasitology). University of Nairobi.

Swallow B. 2000. Impacts of Trypanosomiasis on African Agriculture, Food and Agriculture Organization of the United Nations, Roma.

Tanenbe C, Gambo H, Musongong AG, Boris O, Achukwi MD. 2010. Prévalence de la trypanosomose bovine dans les départements du Faro et Déo, et de la Vina au Cameroun : bilan de vingt années de lutte contre les glossines. Revue d'élevage et de médecine vétérinaire des pays tropicaux, 63 (3-4), 63-69

Taioe M, Makhosazanay MBN, Amos C. 2017. Characterisation of tabanid flies (Diptera: Tabanidae) in South Africa and Zambia and detection of protozoans parasites they are harbouring. Parasitology, 144 (9), 1162-1178.

Thrusfield, M. 2007. Veterinary epidemiology. 3rd Edition. Blackwell, Oxford, UK. 610 pages.

Vall E, Bayala I. 2004. Note d'état corporel des zébus soudaniens. Fiche technique n° 12, CIRDES. 8 pages.

Wells EA. 1972. The importance of mechanical transmission in the epidemiology of nagana : A review. Tropical Animal Health and Production, 4, 74-88.

Woudamyata AF. 2014. Contrôle de la trypanosomose bovine par l'utilisation de la cypermethrine 3 % en "pour-on" dans la zone infestée du Faro et Deo. In Mémoire présenté en vue de l'obtention du diplôme de docteur en médecine vétérinaire. Ecole des sciences et de médecine vétérinaire, Université de Ngaoundéré, Cameroun. 82 pages.

Zumpt F. 1973. The Stomoxyinae biting flies of the world. Taxonomy, biology, economic Importance and control measures. Gustav Fischer Verlag, Stuttgart, 175pp.

www.ingramcontent.com/pod-product-compliance
Lightning Source LLC
Chambersburg PA
CBHW040902110726
48005CB00001B/167